Modern HIV Prevention, Made Simple

PrEP and Doxy-PEP for Sexual Health Protection

Vanesha Goffe, DNP, AAHIVS

Copyright

Table Of Contents

Medical Disclaimer

The information provided in this book is for educational purposes only and is not intended as medical advice. The content reflects current public health guidance and clinical evidence at the time of publication.

This book does not establish a provider–patient relationship and should not be used as a substitute for professional medical consultation, diagnosis, or treatment.

Readers should consult a qualified healthcare provider regarding individual medical decisions, including HIV prevention strategies, PrEP initiation, Doxy-PEP use, laboratory monitoring, and risk assessment.

Clinical guidelines evolve. Recommendations may change over time as new evidence emerges.

The author makes no representations or warranties regarding specific outcomes and disclaims liability for any adverse effects resulting from the use or application of information contained in this publication.

Dedication

This book is dedicated to the communities disproportionately impacted by HIV, to clinicians committed to prevention equity, and to every patient who deserves access to evidence-based, stigma-free sexual healthcare.

It is also dedicated to my family, whose love, patience, and support carried me through the long days, late nights, and sacrifices required to complete this work. Thank you for understanding the time I spent while pursuing this vision and for always encouraging me to keep going.

Introduction

HIV prevention has changed dramatically over the past decade. We now have highly effective tools that can prevent HIV and reduce the burden of other sexually transmitted infections (STIs). Yet new HIV infections continue to occur, particularly among young adults and communities that already face barriers to healthcare access.

This book is not here to judge your choices, label your behavior, or tell you how to live your life. It's here to make sure you have access to accurate information so you can make decisions that feel right for you and close gaps.

As a clinician working in primary care and sexual health, I have witnessed firsthand how often HIV prevention opportunities are missed, not because patients do not care about their health, but because conversations never happen, information is incomplete, or systems make prevention difficult to access. Many people still believe HIV prevention is "not for them," or they are unsure how to ask for protection without fear of judgment.

This guide is intentionally **judgment-free, patient-centered, and practical**. It does not assume risk, identity, or behavior. Instead, it focuses on exposing what situations create vulnerability and how modern prevention tools can be used safely, responsibly, and effectively.

You will find clear explanations of:

- Pre-exposure prophylaxis (PrEP) for HIV prevention
- Doxycycline post-exposure prophylaxis (Doxy-PEP) for selected bacterial STIs

- How to assess exposure without stigma
- How to build a layered prevention plan that fits real life
- How clinicians, clinics, and health departments can implement prevention consistently

This book is written for **everyone**:

- individuals seeking to protect their sexual health,
- clinicians wanting practical, evidence-based guidance, and
- Public health professionals are working to expand prevention access.

You do not need to read this book cover to cover. Some readers may focus on personal prevention options, while others may use case-based and implementation chapters as tools for practice. Each chapter includes reflection questions to support learning, discussion, and system improvement.

Prevention works best when information is accessible, conversations are normalized, and care is delivered without judgment. My hope is that this book empowers you to ask questions, explore options, and participate actively in protecting your health or the health of the communities you serve.

About the Author

Vanesha Goffe, DNP, MSN-Ed, FNP-BC, APRN, AAHIVS, is a doctoral-prepared Family Nurse Practitioner with clinical expertise in HIV prevention and sexual health.

She holds the AAHIVS credential (American Academy of HIV Medicine HIV Specialist), a nationally recognized certification awarded to clinicians who demonstrate specialized knowledge and competency in the prevention, diagnosis, and management of HIV. This designation reflects focused training and ongoing education in evidence-based HIV care.

Dr. Goffe's clinical practice emphasizes exposure-based prevention, PrEP integration, Doxy-PEP education, and equitable access to sexual health services. Her passion for HIV prevention grew from witnessing preventable infections in young adults and underserved communities, reinforcing the importance of proactive, informed prevention strategies.

She is committed to translating complex clinical evidence into clear, practical guidance that empowers both patients and providers. Her work is rooted in a simple belief: prevention works when information is accessible, conversations are normalized, and systems support consistent care.

Author's Note:

"This book is my way of giving readers the tools, knowledge, and confidence to take control of their sexual health without judgment, fear, or shame. Everyone deserves access to prevention, and my hope is that these pages empower you to protect yourself and live confidently."

Professional inquiries: goffehealthandwellness@gmail.com

How to Use This Book

This guide is designed to support both clinicians and individuals seeking a clear, practical understanding of modern HIV prevention strategies. It provides evidence-based, easy-to-apply information on pre-exposure prophylaxis (PrEP), post-exposure prophylaxis with doxycycline (Doxy-PEP), and comprehensive sexual health care.

For Clinicians

Clinicians can use this guide as a quick reference to:
- Identify appropriate candidates for PrEP
- Initiate PrEP safely and efficiently
- Apply recommended laboratory monitoring
- Integrate HIV prevention into routine primary care practice
- Provide patient-centered counseling and risk-reduction strategies

Clinical tables, appendices, and quick-reference sections are included to support real-time decision-making in practice settings.

For Patients and the General Public

This guide also serves as an educational resource for individuals seeking to better understand HIV prevention. It explains prevention options in clear, accessible language and empowers readers to engage in informed discussions with their healthcare providers.

How to Navigate This Guide

- Early chapters provide foundational knowledge on HIV prevention strategies
- Clinical sections offer structured guidance for implementation
- Appendices include quick-reference tools for laboratory testing and monitoring

- Clinical pearls highlight key takeaways for practical
application
Readers may use this guide sequentially or refer to specific
sections based on their needs

Clinical Update Statement

This guide reflects current clinical recommendations at the time
of publication. HIV prevention strategies, including PrEP
modalities and laboratory monitoring, continue to evolve.
Clinicians are encouraged to integrate emerging evidence,
updated guidelines, and clinical judgment into practice.

Quick Prevention Summary

HIV is preventable.

• PrEP (pre-exposure prophylaxis) can reduce the risk of sexual
HIV acquisition by up to 99% when taken as prescribed.
• Doxy-PEP (doxycycline post-exposure prophylaxis) can reduce
the risk of some bacterial STIs, especially syphilis and
chlamydia, when taken soon after exposure in appropriately
selected individuals.

Prevention works best when it is layered:
• Routine HIV testing
• Routine STI screening and treatment
• PrEP when HIV exposure is possible
• Doxy-PEP when recurrent bacterial STIs and ongoing exposure
risk make it appropriate
• Condoms as a risk-reduction tool
• Vaccines (e.g., hepatitis B, HPV)
• Harm reduction supports (e.g., syringe services, substance-use
treatment)

If your clinic visit includes STI treatment or HIV testing, it is
appropriate to ask: "Can we talk about prevention options like
PrEP or Doxy-PEP?"

Chapter 1

The Prevention Paradox: Why HIV Persists in the Era of Effective Intervention

HIV is a preventable infection.

Pre-exposure prophylaxis (PrEP) reduces the risk of sexual HIV acquisition by up to 99% when taken as prescribed (CDC, 2023; USPSTF, 2023). Advances in antiretroviral therapy have transformed HIV into a manageable chronic condition for many individuals. Diagnostic testing is widely available, and public health prevention frameworks are well established.

Despite these advances, new HIV diagnoses continue to occur each year in the United States and globally (CDC, 2023; World Health Organization [WHO], 2022).

This represents a prevention paradox.

The persistence of HIV transmission is not primarily due to pharmacologic failure. It reflects gaps in implementation.

These gaps include:

- Inconsistent routine exposure screening
- Limited proactive offering of PrEP
- Structural barriers to access
- Stigma surrounding sexual health conversations
- Health system fragmentation

The biomedical tools exist. The systems supporting their use are inconsistent.

From Identity-Based to Exposure-Based Prevention

Historically, HIV prevention efforts have been closely associated with identity categories. While epidemiologic patterns may identify disproportionately affected communities, clinical decision-making must be guided by exposure risk rather than identity, empowering providers and patients to take control of prevention.

Exposure-based prevention evaluates behaviors and contexts, including:

- Number and type of sexual partners
- Condom use patterns
- History of sexually transmitted bacterial infections
- Partner HIV status
- Injection drug use practices

When prevention is offered only to individuals who "appear high risk," missed opportunities are inevitable.

Routine, standardized exposure assessment reduces bias and normalizes prevention.

Implementation Failures in Practice

In many healthcare settings, HIV testing is offered, but prevention counseling is not integrated into the workflow.

For example:

A patient presenting with recurrent bacterial STIs may receive treatment without documentation of a PrEP discussion. An individual with a partner living with HIV may not be informed about preventive options unless they initiate the conversation.

These patterns reflect system-level gaps rather than patient-level failure.

From a public health standpoint, effective prevention requires:

- Standardized screening protocols
- Routine PrEP offering when indicated
- Integration of STI and HIV prevention services
- Addressing insurance and cost barriers

Without these elements, prevention remains reactive rather than proactive.

The Role of Stigma in Prevention Gaps

Stigma remains a structural barrier.

Sexual health conversations are often avoided in clinical encounters due to discomfort, time constraints, or assumptions. Patients may hesitate to disclose exposure risk due to fear of judgment.

Stigma functions as a systems issue rather than a personal failing. When prevention conversations are normalized, uptake improves.

Reducing stigma is not an abstract moral goal. It is a measurable public health intervention.

A Public Health Reframing

Modern HIV prevention requires a shift in framing:

Not:
Who is at risk?

But:
What exposures are occurring? This shift from asking, 'Who is at risk?' to 'What exposures are occurring?' aims to empower clinicians to make precise, effective prevention decisions, fostering confidence in their role in reducing HIV transmission.

Not:
Does this patient identify with a high-risk group?

But:
Would biomedical prevention reduce the risk of transmission in this context?

This reframing aligns prevention with exposure science rather than social categorization.

Chapter Summary

HIV persists not because prevention tools are ineffective, but because implementation is inconsistent.

Effective prevention requires:

- Routine exposure-based screening
- Proactive offering of biomedical tools
- Integration of STI and HIV services
- Addressing structural barriers
- Normalization of sexual health conversations

The goal is not rhetorical advocacy. The goal is clinical precision and systems alignment.

Reflection

Clinical Reflection

- Is exposure screening standardized in my setting?
- Are PrEP discussions routinely initiated when indicated?
- Where are prevention opportunities being missed?

Individual Reflection

- Have I discussed prevention options with a provider?
- What exposures in my life warrant a prevention conversation?

Systems Consideration

- Are prevention services accessible and affordable in my community?
- What institutional policies could improve prevention integration?

Chapter 2

Exposure-Based Risk Assessment: Reframing HIV Prevention

Introduction

Effective HIV prevention begins with accurate risk assessment.

Historically, prevention efforts have often relied on identity-based assumptions. While epidemiologic data may demonstrate disproportionate impact among certain populations, clinical decision-making must be guided by exposure risk rather than demographic labels.

Exposure-based risk assessment focuses on behaviors, contexts, and biological vulnerability rather than identity categories. This shift is essential to reducing missed prevention opportunities and normalizing prevention conversations (Centers for Disease Control and Prevention [CDC], 2023).

This chapter outlines the principles of exposure-based assessment and its role in modern HIV and STI prevention.

Why Identity-Based Screening Falls Short

Epidemiological surveillance helps identify population-level disparities. However, translating those patterns into individual-level screening decisions can introduce bias.

When providers rely on perceived identity rather than exposure patterns, several problems may occur:

- Individuals outside traditionally recognized groups may not be offered prevention.
- Assumptions may replace direct, structured assessment.
- Patients may feel labeled or judged.

The U.S. Preventive Services Task Force (USPSTF, 2023) recommends offering PrEP based on exposure-related risk factors rather than identity alone. Routine assessment improves prevention equity.

Exposure does not require a label. It requires evaluation.

Defining Exposure-Based Risk

Exposure-based risk assessment evaluates factors such as:

- Number and type of sexual partners
- Consistency of condom use
- History of sexually transmitted bacterial infections
- Partner HIV status
- Use of injection drugs or shared equipment

Recurrent bacterial STIs are a particularly strong indicator of ongoing exposure risk (CDC, 2023).

Exposure-based assessment should occur routinely in:

- Primary care visits
- STI treatment encounters
- College health settings
- Community clinics
- Public health programs

Risk assessment is not a one-time event. Exposure patterns may change over time.

Normalizing Routine Screening

Routine screening reduces stigma.

When exposure assessment is universal rather than selective, patients are less likely to feel targeted. Prevention becomes part of standard healthcare rather than a specialized intervention.

For example:

Instead of asking,
"Are you at high risk for HIV?"

A provider may ask,
"Have you had any new sexual partners in the past six months?"

The second question is neutral, structured, and exposure-focused.

Standardization improves consistency and reduces implicit bias.

Missed Opportunities in Clinical Practice

Despite clear guidance, exposure assessment is inconsistently implemented.

Studies show that PrEP remains underprescribed relative to eligibility, particularly among women, heterosexual individuals, and racial and ethnic minority populations (USPSTF, 2023; CDC, 2023).

Common gaps include:

- STI treatment visits without prevention discussion

- HIV testing without PrEP counseling
- Time constraints limiting structured screening
- Provider discomfort discussing sexual health

These gaps are implementation challenges, not pharmacologic limitations.

Clinical Vignette

A 29-year-old patient presents for treatment of gonorrhea. This is the second documented STI in 12 months. HIV testing is negative.

The visit concludes with antibiotic treatment and discharge instructions. No documentation reflects discussion of PrEP eligibility.

From a systems perspective, this represents a missed opportunity for prevention.

An exposure-based framework would identify recurrent STIs as an indicator of ongoing HIV exposure risk and trigger a structured prevention conversation.

Integrating Exposure Assessment into Workflow

Exposure-based screening should be:

- Standardized
- Brief
- Routine
- Documented

Simple screening prompts may include:

- "Have you had any new sexual partners since your last visit?"
- "Do you know the HIV status of your partners?"
- "Have you had any STIs in the past year?"
- "Do you inject drugs or share equipment?"

Documentation ensures continuity of care and enables proactive follow-up.

For public health settings, integrating screening tools into intake forms can increase consistency.

Addressing Patient Concerns

Patients may hesitate to disclose exposure due to fear of judgment.

Clear messaging improves transparency:

"Everyone is asked these questions so we can offer prevention options when appropriate."

This normalizes assessment and reinforces routine care.

Exposure-based conversations should focus on health protection rather than risk labeling.

Public Health Impact

Shifting to exposure-based prevention improves:

- Prevention equity
- PrEP uptake
- Early intervention
- STI control
- HIV incidence reduction

Population-level reductions depend on consistent application of exposure assessment across clinical settings (CDC, 2023).

Without structured screening, prevention remains reactive.

Chapter Summary

Exposure-based risk assessment is the foundation of modern HIV prevention.

It shifts focus from identity to behavior and context.

Effective implementation requires:

- Routine, standardized screening
- Neutral, structured language
- Documentation and follow-up
- Integration into STI and primary care visits

Prevention improves when exposure assessment is normalized and consistent.

Reflection

Clinical Reflection

- Is exposure screening standardized in my practice?
- Are recurrent STIs triggering prevention discussions?
- Is documentation consistent?

Individual Reflection

- Have I been asked structured exposure questions during healthcare visits?
- Have I disclosed exposure patterns honestly?
- Do I understand how exposure influences prevention options?

Systems Consideration

- Are screening tools integrated into intake processes?
- Are there workflow barriers limiting prevention conversations?
- Are prevention services equitably offered across populations?

Chapter 3

Pre-Exposure Prophylaxis (PrEP): Evidence, Indications, Safety, and Public Health Impact

Introduction

Pre-exposure prophylaxis (PrEP) is one of the most effective biomedical strategies available for preventing HIV acquisition. When taken as prescribed, PrEP reduces the risk of sexual HIV transmission by up to 99% (Centers for Disease Control and Prevention [CDC], 2023; U.S. Preventive Services Task Force [USPSTF], 2023).

PrEP represents a shift from reactive HIV treatment to proactive prevention. Rather than waiting for exposure to occur, PrEP provides pharmacologic protection before HIV transmission can take place.

This chapter reviews the evidence base, eligibility criteria, safety considerations, and public health implications of PrEP.

The Evidence Base

PrEP efficacy has been demonstrated in multiple large randomized controlled trials.

The iPrEx trial showed that daily oral tenofovir-based PrEP significantly reduced HIV acquisition among men who have sex with men (Grant et al., 2010).

Subsequent trials demonstrated similar efficacy in heterosexual men and women (Baeten et al., 2012).

Long-acting injectable formulations have also shown high efficacy in preventing HIV acquisition in at-risk populations (Landovitz et al., 2021).

Real-world implementation studies further confirm that adherence is strongly correlated with protection. When taken consistently, PrEP provides near-complete protection against sexual HIV acquisition (CDC, 2023).

Who Should Be Offered PrEP?

PrEP eligibility is based on exposure risk rather than identity. However, providers may need guidance on identifying at-risk populations, such as those with multiple partners or inconsistent condom use, to ensure appropriate prescribing.

According to USPSTF recommendations (2023), PrEP should be offered to individuals who:

- Have a sexual partner living with HIV
- Have had a recent bacterial STI
- Have multiple sexual partners with inconsistent condom use
- Engage in transactional sex
- Inject drugs and share equipment

Routine exposure screening normalizes prevention and reduces missed opportunities.

PrEP should not be limited to individuals who identify with specific demographic groups. Clinical assessment should focus on exposure patterns.

Available PrEP Options

Daily Oral PrEP

Daily oral tenofovir-based regimens remain widely used and effective.

Advantages:

- Established safety profile
- Familiarity among clinicians
- Broad insurance coverage

Considerations:

- Requires daily adherence
- Requires routine laboratory monitoring

Long-Acting Injectable PrEP

Long-acting injectable PrEP is administered at scheduled intervals by a healthcare provider.

Advantages:

- Eliminates daily pill burden
- May improve adherence
- Reduces reliance on patient memory

Considerations:

- Requires clinic visits
- May present access or cost barriers

The choice of regimen should be individualized based on patient preferences, access, and clinical considerations.

Baseline Evaluation and Monitoring

Before initiating PrEP, clinicians should:

- Confirm negative HIV status
- Assess renal function
- Screen for hepatitis B
- Conduct baseline STI testing

Ongoing monitoring typically includes:

- HIV testing every 3 months
- Renal function monitoring (for oral PrEP)
- Routine STI screening

For patients, this means PrEP involves regular follow-up, not a one-time prescription.

Monitoring ensures both safety and early detection of potential HIV seroconversion.

Safety and Tolerability

PrEP is generally well-tolerated.

Common side effects may include:

- Mild gastrointestinal symptoms
- Headache
- Transient fatigue

Renal effects are rare but require monitoring in oral formulations (CDC, 2023).

Long-acting injectable formulations may cause injection site reactions, typically mild.

Overall, PrEP has demonstrated a strong safety profile across diverse populations.

Public Health Impact

PrEP is a cornerstone of national HIV prevention strategies.

Widespread PrEP uptake has been associated with reductions in HIV incidence in communities with strong implementation efforts (CDC, 2023).

However, uptake remains uneven. Barriers include:

- Cost and insurance limitations
- Stigma
- Lack of provider awareness
- Misinformation

Public health success depends on the routine offering of PrEP when indicated, rather than relying on patient self-advocacy alone.

Clinical Vignette

A 24-year-old patient presents for routine STI testing. They report multiple partners over the past year and inconsistent condom use. HIV testing is negative.

Rather than limiting the screening visit, the clinician discusses PrEP eligibility based on exposure risk. After reviewing benefits, monitoring requirements, and potential side effects, the patient elects to initiate PrEP.

This interaction reflects proactive prevention rather than reactive testing alone.

Addressing Common Misconceptions

PrEP does not treat HIV.
It prevents HIV acquisition.

PrEP does not protect against all STIs.
It specifically reduces HIV risk.

PrEP is not limited to any one population.
Eligibility is determined by exposure risk.

Chapter Summary

PrEP is a highly effective, evidence-supported HIV prevention strategy.

When taken as prescribed, it reduces HIV acquisition risk by up to 99%.

Appropriate implementation requires:

- Exposure-based screening
- Baseline evaluation
- Routine monitoring
- Patient education
- Access support

Expanding routine PrEP offering remains essential to reducing HIV incidence.

Reflection

Clinical Reflection

- Is PrEP routinely offered when exposure risk is identified?
- Are monitoring protocols standardized in practice?
- Are assumptions influencing eligibility discussions?

Individual Reflection

- Is HIV exposure possible in my life?
- Have I discussed PrEP with a provider?
- What barriers might prevent access?

Systems Consideration

- Are cost and insurance barriers limiting uptake?
- Is provider education sufficient in my community?
- Are prevention conversations normalized in clinical settings?

Chapter 4

PrEP Monitoring, Adherence, and Access

Introduction

Pre-exposure prophylaxis (PrEP) is highly effective when taken as prescribed. However, efficacy depends on appropriate initiation, monitoring, adherence support, and continuity of access.

PrEP is not a single prescription event. It is a structured prevention intervention requiring ongoing clinical oversight (Centers for Disease Control and Prevention [CDC], 2023; U.S. Preventive Services Task Force [USPSTF], 2023).

This chapter outlines the clinical monitoring framework, safety considerations, adherence factors, and access barriers relevant to successful PrEP implementation.

Baseline Evaluation Before Initiation

Before starting PrEP, clinicians should:

- Confirm negative HIV status using appropriate testing
- Assess renal function (for oral tenofovir-based regimens)
- Screen for hepatitis B infection
- Conduct baseline STI testing
- Evaluate pregnancy potential when applicable

Confirming HIV-negative status prior to initiation is essential to avoid resistance development if acute HIV infection is present (CDC, 2023).

Baseline assessment ensures both safety and appropriate candidacy.

Ongoing Monitoring

Once initiated, PrEP requires regular follow-up.

Typical monitoring includes:

- HIV testing every 2–3 months
- Renal function monitoring for oral regimens
- STI screening at regular intervals
- Assessment of adherence and side effects

Monitoring protects both individual health and public health integrity.

Regular HIV testing ensures early detection in the rare event of seroconversion while on PrEP.

Safety Profile

PrEP has a strong safety record across diverse populations.

Common side effects may include:

- Mild gastrointestinal symptoms
- Headache
- Fatigue

For oral tenofovir-based regimens, small changes in renal function may occur but are typically reversible upon discontinuation (CDC, 2023).

Long-acting injectable PrEP may cause injection site reactions, usually mild and transient (Landovitz et al., 2021).

Overall, serious adverse effects are uncommon.

Risk–benefit assessment consistently favors PrEP use in individuals with meaningful exposure risk.

Adherence and Effectiveness

Adherence strongly correlates with protection.

Clinical trials demonstrate that protective drug levels significantly reduce HIV acquisition risk (Grant et al., 2010; Baeten et al., 2012).

Missed doses reduce effectiveness but do not immediately eliminate protection. Counseling should emphasize consistency rather than perfection.

For patients:

PrEP works best when taken as prescribed. If doses are missed, providers should discuss strategies to improve adherence rather than discontinue therapy reflexively.

For clinicians:

Routine adherence assessment should be structured and nonjudgmental.

Addressing Barriers to Continuation

Common barriers to PrEP continuation include:

- Cost concerns
- Insurance changes
- Transportation challenges
- Stigma
- Pill fatigue

Discontinuation often reflects structural issues rather than a lack of motivation.

Strategies to improve retention include:

- Clear explanation of assistance programs
- Flexible appointment scheduling
- Telehealth options
- Reminder systems
- Integration with primary care

Prevention continuity requires proactive follow-up.

Access and Insurance Considerations

Although PrEP is recommended by the USPSTF (2023), coverage varies across plans and states.

Barriers may include:

- Prior authorization requirements
- Limited coverage for long-acting injectable formulations
- Laboratory testing costs
- Pharmacy access limitations

Health departments and community clinics play an important role in facilitating access through:

- Medication assistance programs
- Federally qualified health centers
- Public funding mechanisms
- Community outreach

Simplifying access improves uptake and continuity.

Clinical Vignette

A 31-year-old patient initiates daily oral PrEP but misses follow-up visits due to work schedule conflicts. They report difficulty attending quarterly appointments.

Rather than discontinuing PrEP, the clinic transitions the patient to telehealth follow-up with laboratory coordination at a local facility.

Prevention continuity improves when systems adapt to patient needs.

When to Pause or Discontinue PrEP

PrEP may be paused or discontinued when:

- Exposure risk has decreased
- Renal function concerns arise
- Patient preference changes

Discontinuation decisions should be exposure-based rather than assumption-based.

If exposure risk resumes, PrEP can be restarted with appropriate evaluation.

Prevention should be dynamic.

Public Health Implications

PrEP monitoring and adherence support are essential components of national HIV prevention strategies (CDC, 2023).

High uptake without continuity limits population-level impact.

Successful implementation depends on:

- Standardized protocols
- Ongoing education
- Access support
- Structured follow-up

Monitoring is not an administrative burden. It is prevention integrity.

Chapter Summary

PrEP is safe and highly effective when appropriately monitored.

Successful implementation requires:

- Baseline evaluation
- Routine HIV testing
- Renal monitoring (for oral regimens)
- STI screening
- Adherence support
- Access facilitation

Prevention effectiveness depends not only on medication efficacy but also on continuity and structured oversight.

Reflection

Clinical Reflection

- Are baseline and follow-up protocols standardized?
- Is adherence assessed routinely and constructively?
- Are discontinuation decisions exposure-based?

Individual Reflection

- Do I understand the monitoring schedule for PrEP?
- What barriers might affect my ability to continue?
- Have I discussed adherence challenges openly?

Systems Consideration

- Are cost and laboratory fees limiting retention?
- Is follow-up flexible and accessible?

Chapter 5

Doxycycline Post-Exposure Prophylaxis (Doxy-PEP): Evidence, Indications, and Public Health Considerations

Introduction

Bacterial sexually transmitted infections (STIs), including syphilis, chlamydia, and gonorrhea, have increased substantially in recent years in the United States (Centers for Disease Control and Prevention, 2023). Recurrent infections contribute to ongoing transmission networks and may increase biological susceptibility to HIV acquisition.

Doxycycline post-exposure prophylaxis (Doxy-PEP) is an emerging biomedical strategy designed to reduce the incidence of certain bacterial STIs following sexual exposure. Unlike pre-exposure prophylaxis (PrEP), which is taken prior to potential HIV exposure, Doxy-PEP is administered after a sexual encounter.

This chapter reviews the evidence base, appropriate clinical use, safety considerations, and public health implications of Doxy-PEP.

The Evidence Base

Doxycycline has long been used to treat bacterial STIs. Its use as post-exposure prophylaxis has been evaluated in randomized controlled trials.

In a landmark randomized study, doxycycline taken within 72 hours after sexual exposure significantly reduced the incidence of syphilis and chlamydia among men who have sex with men (Molina et al., 2015).

More recently, a large, randomized trial demonstrated that Doxy-PEP reduced the incidence of:

- Syphilis
- Chlamydia
- Some gonorrhea infections

among individuals at elevated risk for recurrent STIs (Luetkemeyer et al., 2023).

Reductions were substantial for syphilis and chlamydia. The reduction in gonorrhea was more modest, likely due to preexisting tetracycline resistance in certain strains (Luetkemeyer et al., 2023).

From a public health perspective, reducing recurrent bacterial STIs may:

- Interrupt transmission chains
- Decrease inflammatory conditions that increase HIV susceptibility
- Reduce healthcare utilization related to repeated infections

Indications and Appropriate Candidates

Doxy-PEP is not intended for universal use.

Current evidence supports consideration in individuals who:

- Have a documented history of recurrent bacterial STIs
- Are at ongoing sexual exposure risk
- Can adhere to post-exposure timing recommendations
- Understanding antimicrobial stewardship principles

Clinical judgment remains essential. Risk–benefit assessment should consider:

- Frequency of exposure
- History of recurrent infections
- Local resistance patterns
- Ability to follow monitoring recommendations

Doxy-PEP should be discussed as part of a comprehensive prevention strategy rather than as a standalone intervention.

Dosing and Timing

Doxy-PEP is typically administered as a single 200 mg dose of doxycycline taken within 72 hours following condomless sexual exposure (Luetkemeyer et al., 2023).

It is not intended for continuous daily use unless specifically indicated.

Clear patient education is essential. Instructions should include:

- Timing of administration
- Avoidance of exceeding the recommended frequency
- Understanding that Doxy-PEP does not prevent HIV
- Continued need for routine STI screening

Safety and Tolerability

Doxycycline is generally well tolerated. Common adverse effects may include:

- Gastrointestinal discomfort
- Photosensitivity
- Esophagitis (particularly if taken without adequate fluid)

Patients should be counseled to:

- Take medication with water
- Avoid lying down immediately after ingestion
- Use sun protection when appropriate

Contraindications include known hypersensitivity to tetracyclines and certain pregnancy considerations.

Antimicrobial Stewardship and Resistance

Antimicrobial resistance is a critical consideration.

The expanded use of antibiotics for prevention raises legitimate concerns regarding:

- Tetracycline-resistant gonorrhea
- Broader microbiome impact
- Long-term resistance patterns

Public health agencies emphasize that Doxy-PEP should be targeted to individuals at the highest risk rather than broadly prescribed (CDC, 2023).

Ongoing surveillance and stewardship frameworks are necessary to balance individual benefit with population-level consequences.

Doxy-PEP implementation should occur within structured clinical oversight, not informal or unsupervised use.

Integration Into Layered Prevention

Doxy-PEP does not replace:

- HIV PrEP
- Condom use
- Routine STI screening
- Risk-reduction counseling

Instead, it may be integrated into a layered prevention model that includes:

- HIV PrEP for HIV prevention
- Doxy-PEP for selected bacterial STI prevention
- Regular testing intervals
- Open provider–patient communication

Prevention is most effective when interventions are combined appropriately.

Clinical Vignette

A 30-year-old patient receiving HIV PrEP presents with two documented episodes of chlamydia and one episode of syphilis within the past 18 months. Condom use is inconsistent. HIV testing remains negative, and adherence to PrEP is confirmed.

Rather than continuing episodic treatment alone, the provider discusses Doxy-PEP as a targeted strategy to reduce the risk of recurrent bacterial STIs.

This represents a shift from reactive treatment to proactive risk reduction.

Public Health Implications

The introduction of Doxy-PEP reflects a broader evolution in STI prevention strategies.

Historically, STI management focused primarily on diagnosis and treatment. Doxy-PEP represents a preventive extension of antimicrobial therapy.

Successful implementation depends on:

- Clear eligibility criteria
- Structured monitoring
- Education on appropriate use
- Integration with existing HIV prevention frameworks

As evidence evolves, guidelines may be updated. Ongoing research will continue to inform best practices.

Chapter Summary

Doxy-PEP is an emerging, evidence-supported strategy that reduces the incidence of certain bacterial STIs when taken within 72 hours following sexual exposure.

It is most appropriate for individuals with recurrent bacterial STIs and ongoing risk of exposure.

Use should be targeted, monitored, and integrated into a layered prevention model that includes HIV PrEP and routine screening.

Balancing individual benefit with antimicrobial stewardship remains essential.

Reflection

Clinical Reflection

- Are patients with recurrent STIs being offered preventive options beyond episodic treatment?
- Is Doxy-PEP discussed within a structured stewardship framework?
- How is resistance surveillance incorporated into decision-making?

Individual Reflection

- Have I experienced recurrent bacterial STIs?
- Have I discussed preventive options beyond treatment?
- Do I understand what Doxy-PEP does and does not prevent?

Systems Consideration

- Are prevention strategies integrated into STI treatment workflows?
- Are access barriers limiting appropriate Doxy-PEP use?
- Is antimicrobial stewardship addressed in local protocols?

Chapter 6

Layered Prevention Frameworks: Integrating Biomedical and Behavioral Strategies

Introduction

No single prevention strategy is sufficient to eliminate HIV and STI transmission at the population level.

Modern HIV prevention requires a layered framework combining biomedical tools, behavioral strategies, routine screening, and structural support. When multiple strategies are used together, overall transmission risk decreases substantially (Centers for Disease Control and Prevention [CDC], 2023).

Layered prevention acknowledges that exposure risk varies over time and that individuals benefit from flexible, individualized approaches.

This chapter outlines the components of layered prevention and how they function together in clinical and public health practice.

The Concept of Layered Prevention

Layered prevention is based on a simple principle:

Risk reduction improves when complementary strategies are combined. Rather than relying solely on one intervention, prevention may include:

- HIV pre-exposure prophylaxis (PrEP)
- Doxycycline post-exposure prophylaxis (Doxy-PEP), when indicated
- Condom use
- Routine HIV and STI testing
- Harm reduction strategies for injection drug use
- Vaccination (e.g., hepatitis B, HPV)

Each component addresses a different transmission pathway.

Biomedical interventions reduce biological susceptibility.
Behavioral strategies reduce exposure probability.
Structural interventions improve access and uptake.

Together, they form a comprehensive prevention framework.

Biomedical Prevention as a Foundation

HIV PrEP

PrEP reduces sexual HIV acquisition risk by up to 99% when taken as prescribed (CDC, 2023; U.S. Preventive Services Task Force [USPSTF], 2023).

PrEP addresses HIV transmission specifically but does not prevent bacterial STIs.

Doxy-PEP

Doxy-PEP reduces the incidence of syphilis and chlamydia when taken within 72 hours of sexual exposure (Luetkemeyer et al., 2023).

Its use should be targeted and guided by antimicrobial stewardship principles.

Biomedical prevention reduces biological risk but does not eliminate exposure behaviors. Layering additional strategies enhances protection.

Behavioral Strategies

Condom Use

Condoms reduce the risk of HIV and many STIs when used consistently and correctly (CDC, 2023).

Although adherence may vary, condoms remain an important protective tool within layered prevention.

Routine Testing

Routine HIV and STI testing allows for:

- Early detection
- Prompt treatment
- Prevention of onward transmission
- Identification of prevention eligibility

Testing intervals depend on exposure risk, typically every 3–6 months for those at ongoing risk (CDC, 2023).

Risk-Reduction Counseling

Structured counseling supports informed decision-making and improves adherence to prevention strategies.

Counseling should focus on:

- Exposure patterns
- Medication adherence
- Timing of Doxy-PEP
- Recognition of symptoms
- Access barriers

Risk-reduction counseling is most effective when integrated into routine care rather than delivered only during crisis moments.

Harm Reduction for Injection Drug Use

For individuals who inject drugs, layered prevention includes:

- Access to sterile injection equipment
- Medication-assisted treatment
- HIV PrEP when indicated
- Routine testing

Syringe services programs have demonstrated effectiveness in reducing HIV transmission among people who inject drugs (CDC, 2023).

Harm reduction is a public health strategy grounded in risk reduction rather than abstinence mandates.

Vaccination as Prevention

Vaccination plays an important role in layered sexual health protection.

Relevant vaccines may include:

- Hepatitis B
- Human papillomavirus (HPV)
- Hepatitis A (in certain populations)

Vaccination reduces the risk of long-term complications and transmission.

Layered prevention extends beyond HIV alone.

Clinical Vignette

A 26-year-old patient on daily oral PrEP reports inconsistent condom use and two recent episodes of chlamydia.

Rather than discontinuing PrEP or relying solely on STI treatment, the clinician discusses:

- Continued PrEP adherence
- Potential eligibility for Doxy-PEP
- Routine quarterly STI testing
- Vaccination status review

The approach integrates multiple strategies rather than substituting one for another.

This illustrates layered prevention in practice.

Dynamic Risk and Flexible Prevention

Exposure risk is not static.

Life circumstances, relationships, and behaviors change over time.

Layered prevention allows flexibility:

- Initiating PrEP during periods of higher exposure
- Discontinuing when risk decreases
- Using Doxy-PEP selectively
- Adjusting testing frequency

Prevention should adapt to exposure patterns rather than remain fixed.

Public Health Implications

Layered prevention strengthens population-level impact.

When biomedical tools are combined with routine screening and structural access, communities experience:

- Reduced HIV incidence
- Lower STI transmission rates
- Earlier detection
- Improved engagement in care

Prevention strategies are most effective when integrated across clinical settings rather than delivered in isolation.

Fragmented approaches limit effectiveness.

Coordinated implementation enhances outcomes.

Chapter Summary

Layered prevention combines biomedical, behavioral, and structural strategies to reduce HIV and STI transmission.

Key components include:

- PrEP for HIV prevention
- Doxy-PEP for selected bacterial STI prevention
- Condom use
- Routine testing
- Harm reduction
- Vaccination

No single strategy is sufficient alone.

Integrated prevention improves individual protection and population health outcomes.

Reflection

Clinical Reflection

- Are prevention strategies offered in combination rather than isolation?
- Are patients with recurrent STIs evaluated for layered options?
- Is follow-up structured and consistent?

Individual Reflection

- Which prevention strategies align with my current exposure patterns?
- Have I considered combining prevention tools?
- Do I understand how each strategy functions?

Systems Consideration

- Are biomedical and behavioral services integrated within my community?
- Are there access barriers limiting layered prevention?
- Is prevention fragmented across programs?

Chapter 7

Communication Without Assumption: How to Talk About Sexual Health

Conversations drive prevention. When clinicians avoid sexual health discussions or when patients avoid asking questions, prevention opportunities are missed.

A Universal Script That Reduces Stigma

Start with normalizing:

"I ask everyone these questions so we can support your health."

This shifts the conversation from judgment to routine care.

Common Questions Patients Can Ask

- "Can we talk about PrEP?"
- "Am I eligible for Doxy-PEP?"
- "How often should I test?"
- "What vaccines should I have?"
- "What will this cost?"

Encourage patients to bring a written list to visits.

Responding to Shame or Fear

When someone says, "I don't want to be judged," the clinician can respond:

"You're doing the right thing by protecting your health. My role is support, not judgment."

A Brief Training Note for Clinics

Train staff on:

• neutral language

• confidentiality reinforcement

• trauma-informed approaches

• culturally responsive care

Communication is part of the prevention infrastructure.

Reflection

Clinical Reflection

• Do your staff have a shared script for sexual health questions?

• Are your questions asked universally?

• Do you document prevention counseling consistently?

Individual Reflection

• What's the hardest question for you to ask a provider—and why?

• What reassurance would help you feel safe discussing sexual health?

Systems Consideration

• Do local systems support privacy (confidential communication, safe billing, teen/young adult protections)?

• Are prevention messages culturally aligned with community needs?

Chapter 8

Structural Barriers and Equity in HIV Prevention

Introduction

HIV prevention is not solely a clinical issue. It is also a structural issue.

Although highly effective biomedical tools exist, access to prevention remains uneven. Disparities in HIV incidence reflect broader inequities in healthcare access, socioeconomic conditions, stigma, and policy environments (Centers for Disease Control and Prevention [CDC], 2023; World Health Organization [WHO], 2022).

Effective prevention requires attention not only to individual behavior, but also to the systems that shape access and opportunity.

This chapter examines structural barriers to HIV and STI prevention and outlines practical strategies for advancing health equity.

Understanding Structural Barriers

Structural barriers are conditions within healthcare systems, policies, and social environments that limit access to services.

Common barriers include:

- Lack of insurance coverage

- High medication costs
- Transportation limitations
- Limited clinic availability
- Inconsistent provider training
- Stigma and discrimination
- Language and cultural barriers

These barriers influence whether individuals are offered prevention, can access medication, and remain engaged in care.

Prevention tools are only effective when accessible.

Disparities in HIV Incidence

HIV incidence in the United States disproportionately affects:

- Racial and ethnic minority communities
- Individuals in the Southern United States
- Young adults
- People with limited access to healthcare (CDC, 2023)

These disparities are not attributable solely to inherent behavioral differences. They reflect:

- Differences in access to preventive services
- Higher community viral load
- Reduced access to insurance
- Geographic care gaps

Public health responses must address these structural contributors.

Insurance and Cost Barriers

Although many PrEP medications are covered by insurance plans, gaps remain.

Barriers may include:

- Prior authorization requirements
- Inconsistent coverage across states
- Lack of awareness of assistance programs
- Coverage disparities for injectable formulations

Even when medication costs are addressed, laboratory testing and clinical visits may create financial obstacles.

Public health programs and health departments play a critical role in expanding access through:

- Medication assistance programs
- Community-based clinics
- Federally qualified health centers
- Outreach initiatives

Access must be simplified to improve uptake.

Stigma as a Structural Issue

Stigma functions at multiple levels:

- Interpersonal (provider–patient interactions)
- Institutional (clinic policies)
- Community (social norms)

When sexual health discussions are avoided or framed as exceptional, patients may hesitate to disclose exposure risk.

Normalization reduces stigma.

Routine, universal exposure screening signals that prevention is standard of care rather than a targeted intervention.

Equity improves when prevention is offered without assumptions.

Geographic Barriers

Rural areas and certain regions face provider shortages and limited access to HIV prevention services.

Telehealth expansion has improved access in some settings, but broadband limitations and licensing restrictions may remain barriers.

Health departments can mitigate geographic gaps by:

- Supporting mobile clinics
- Expanding telehealth infrastructure
- Partnering with community organizations
- Training primary care providers in prevention delivery

Decentralizing prevention services improves reach.

Cultural and Linguistic Considerations

Culturally responsive care improves prevention uptake.

Barriers may include:

- Limited availability of multilingual services
- Mistrust of healthcare institutions
- Historical inequities affecting healthcare engagement

Community partnerships and culturally tailored outreach improve acceptance and adherence.

Prevention must be adaptable to diverse populations.

Clinical Vignette

A 22-year-old uninsured patient expresses interest in PrEP but is concerned about cost. They were previously told that PrEP was "expensive" and not covered.

The clinician connects the patient with a medication assistance program and arranges low-cost laboratory monitoring through a community clinic.

The barrier was not a lack of motivation. It was a lack of navigational support.

Structural barriers often require system-level solutions rather than individual-level correction.

Strategies to Advance Health Equity

Improving prevention equity requires coordinated efforts:

At the Clinical Level

- Routine exposure-based screening
- Clear explanation of assistance programs
- Simplified referral pathways
- Inclusive language in documentation

At the Organizational Level

- Staff training on prevention guidelines
- Standardized screening protocols
- Integration of STI and HIV services
- Outreach to underserved communities

At the Public Health Level

- Funding for prevention programs
- Expanded insurance coverage
- Data-driven resource allocation
- Community engagement partnerships

Health equity improves when prevention is integrated rather than siloed.

Moving From Access to Implementation

Improving access is necessary but not sufficient.

Prevention must also be:

- Routinely offered
- Documented
- Followed up
- Evaluated for effectiveness

Data collection and program evaluation support continuous improvement.

Health departments and clinics benefit from monitoring:

- PrEP uptake rates
- STI recurrence patterns
- Prevention engagement
- Access disparities

Measurement informs strategy.

Chapter Summary

Structural barriers significantly influence HIV and STI prevention outcomes.

Disparities reflect differences in access, insurance coverage, stigma, geographic availability, and systemic inequities.

Advancing health equity requires:

- Routine exposure-based screening
- Simplified access pathways
- Integration of services
- Community partnership
- Data-informed implementation

Prevention improves when systems support consistent access and delivery.

Reflection

Clinical Reflection

- Are assistance programs routinely discussed?
- Are prevention services offered equitably across populations?
- Are documentation and follow-up consistent?

Individual Reflection

- Have cost or access concerns limited prevention engagement?
- Do I know where to seek low-cost prevention services?
- Have I felt comfortable discussing prevention with a provider?

Systems Consideration

- Are prevention services equitably distributed in my community?
- Are insurance policies limiting access?
- Are outreach efforts reaching underserved populations?

Chapter 9

Case-Based Clinical Application: Translating Prevention Into Practice

Introduction

Effective prevention depends not only on knowledge of biomedical tools but on structured clinical application.

Case-based analysis helps clarify how exposure assessment, PrEP eligibility, Doxy-PEP consideration, monitoring, and structural factors interact in real-world settings.

This chapter presents structured clinical scenarios designed to illustrate decision-making within a layered prevention framework.

Each case demonstrates:

- Exposure-based assessment
- Prevention eligibility
- Monitoring considerations
- Structural barriers
- Systems-level implications

Case 1: Recurrent Bacterial STIs in a Patient on PrEP

Presentation

A 28-year-old patient presents for quarterly PrEP follow-up. HIV testing remains negative. Over the past 18 months, they have experienced:

- Two episodes of chlamydia
- One episode of syphilis

They report inconsistent condom use with multiple partners.

Renal function is normal. PrEP adherence is confirmed.

Clinical Assessment

Key considerations:

- HIV risk remains elevated.
- PrEP adherence is protective against HIV.
- Recurrent bacterial STIs suggest ongoing exposure.
- Current prevention plan is incomplete.

According to CDC guidance (2023) and emerging evidence, individuals with recurrent STIs may be candidates for Doxy-PEP in addition to PrEP (Luetkemeyer et al., 2023).

Intervention Plan

Layered strategy:

- Continue daily oral PrEP.

- Initiate structured discussion regarding Doxy-PEP eligibility.
- Reinforce quarterly STI testing.
- Review vaccination status (hepatitis B, HPV).
- Provide adherence counseling.

Systems Consideration

If Doxy-PEP is not available in the clinic, referral pathways should be established.

Missed opportunities occur when STI treatment remains episodic without preventive escalation.

Key Learning Point

Reactive treatment alone is insufficient when exposure remains ongoing. Layered prevention reduces cumulative risk.

Case 2: Young Adult with New Exposure Risk

Presentation

A 22-year-old college student presents for STI screening. They report:

- A new sexual partner within the past month
- Uncertain partner HIV status
- Inconsistent condom use
- No prior STI history

The HIV test is negative.

Clinical Assessment

Exposure-based screening indicates potential HIV acquisition risk.

Even without prior STIs, eligibility criteria for PrEP may be met (USPSTF, 2023).

Risk assessment should focus on:

- Current exposure
- Anticipated future exposure
- Patient preference

Intervention Plan

- Discuss PrEP as a preventive option.
- Explain the monitoring schedule.
- Review side effect profile.
- Assess insurance coverage.
- Offer initiation if the patient elects.

Doxy-PEP is not indicated without a recurrent STI history or elevated bacterial STI risk.

Systems Consideration

College health settings should integrate exposure screening into routine visits rather than waiting for STI recurrence.

Key Learning Point

Prevention should not be delayed until after infection occurs.

Case 3: Patient Concerned About Cost

Presentation

A 30-year-old uninsured patient expresses interest in PrEP but reports inability to afford medication or laboratory testing.

They have:

- A partner living with HIV
- No insurance coverage
- Limited transportation

Clinical Assessment

Exposure risk is significant.

Barrier: structural, not motivational.

Prevention eligibility is clear, but access is constrained.

Intervention Plan

- Connect the patient with medication assistance programs.
- Coordinate laboratory services through community clinics.
- Explore telehealth options.
- Schedule structured follow-up.

Public health resources often bridge coverage gaps (CDC, 2023).

Systems Consideration

Prevention uptake declines when navigation support is absent.

Access infrastructure is part of the effectiveness of prevention.

Key Learning Point

Structural barriers must be addressed alongside clinical eligibility.

Case 4: Considering Discontinuation of PrEP

Presentation

A 35-year-old patient has been on PrEP for two years. They report entering a mutually monogamous relationship with a partner confirmed HIV-negative.

They request discontinuation.

Clinical Assessment

Exposure risk appears reduced.

Guidelines support discontinuation when risk decreases (CDC, 2023).

However, shared decision-making is essential.

Intervention Plan

- Confirm partner HIV status.
- Discuss window periods and retesting.
- Explain re-initiation procedures if exposure changes.
- Document decision and follow-up plan.

Systems Consideration

Prevention must be dynamic and adaptable.

Rigid continuation without exposure risk may reduce trust in adherence.

Key Learning Point

PrEP decisions should be exposure-based rather than permanent mandates.

Case 5: Gonorrhea Resistance Concerns and Doxy-PEP

Presentation

A 33-year-old patient eligible for Doxy-PEP expresses concern about antibiotic resistance.

They have had:

- Three bacterial STIs in one year
- Ongoing exposure risk
- Strong adherence to PrEP

Clinical Assessment

Doxy-PEP significantly reduces syphilis and chlamydia incidence (Luetkemeyer et al., 2023).

Gonorrhea reduction may be variable due to tetracycline resistance patterns.

Antimicrobial stewardship principles apply.

Intervention Plan

- Discuss benefits and limitations.
- Emphasize targeted use.

- Reinforce routine testing.
- Monitor for recurrent infection.

Systems Consideration

Doxy-PEP should be offered selectively under structured oversight rather than prescribed broadly.

Balancing individual benefit and resistance concerns is essential.

Key Learning Point

Evidence supports the use of targeted Doxy-PEP in high-risk individuals under clinical monitoring.

Integrating Lessons Across Cases

Across these scenarios, consistent themes emerge:

- Exposure assessment drives eligibility.
- Prevention should be layered.
- Monitoring protects safety and public health.
- Structural barriers influence uptake.
- Decisions should be individualized.

Case-based application reinforces that prevention is not a one-size-fits-all model.

Chapter Summary

Translating prevention into practice requires:

- Structured exposure-based assessment
- Evidence-guided eligibility determination
- Layered prevention strategies
- Ongoing monitoring
- Addressing structural barriers
- Shared decision-making

Case-based reasoning clarifies how biomedical prevention functions within real-world contexts.

Effective prevention depends on consistent, structured implementation.

Reflection

Clinical Reflection

- Are recurrent STIs triggering preventive escalation?
- Are cost barriers proactively addressed?
- Are discontinuation decisions exposure-based?

Individual Reflection

- Have I discussed prevention beyond testing?
- Do I understand my eligibility for PrEP or Doxy-PEP?
- What barriers affect my prevention of access?

Systems Consideration

- Are case-based decision tools integrated into training?
- Are referral pathways clear?
- Is prevention offered proactively across settings?

Chapter 10

Doxy-PEP in Real Life: Detailed Q&A, Safety, and Practical

Scenarios

This chapter is dedicated to Doxy-PEP questions because patients and clinicians need clear, practical guidance.

Below are common patient questions with straightforward answers, followed by real-world examples and safety reminders.

Patient Q&A (Clear Answers)

Q: What is Doxy-PEP?
A: Doxy-PEP is doxycycline taken after sexual exposure to reduce the risk of certain bacterial STIs, especially syphilis and chlamydia, in selected individuals.

Q: Does it prevent HIV?
A: No. PrEP is for HIV prevention. Doxy-PEP is for some bacterial STIs.

Q: When do I take it?
A: Many protocols use 200 mg as soon as possible after exposure and within 72 hours. Follow your clinician's instructions.

Q: Can I take it every day?
A: Doxy-PEP is typically not prescribed as a daily medication. It should be used in a targeted way based on eligibility and a prevention plan.

Q: What side effects should I watch for?
A: GI upset, nausea, sun sensitivity, and irritation of the esophagus if taken without water or right before lying down.

Q: Will it make antibiotics stop working?
A: Overuse of antibiotics can contribute to resistance. That's why Doxy-PEP should be targeted and paired with routine testing and reassessment.

Practical Examples

Example 1: Recurrent chlamydia
A patient has two chlamydia infections in a year. They have ongoing exposure risk. The clinician discusses layered prevention: PrEP if HIV exposure is possible, routine testing, vaccines, and whether Doxy-PEP is appropriate.

Example 2: Concern about stigma
A patient worries that Doxy-PEP implies "bad behavior." The clinician reframes: "This is prevention, like a seatbelt. It's not judgment."

Example 3: Medication timing challenge
A patient has trouble remembering. The clinician provides written instructions, a reminder plan, and schedules follow-up testing.

Safety Checklist for Patients

- Take with water.
- Stay upright 30 minutes.
- Use sunscreen.
- Tell your provider about pregnancy possibility, allergies, and other meds.
- Keep routine STI testing.
- Reassess whether you still need Doxy-PEP over time.

Clinician Notes: Stewardship in Practice

Use targeted eligibility, document shared decision-making, track outcomes, and reassess ongoing need. Reinforce that Doxy-PEP is one part of a layered prevention plan.

Reflection

Clinical Reflection

• Do you provide written dosing instructions and side-effect guidance for Doxy-PEP?

• Do you track STI recurrence after initiation and reassess ongoing need?

• Do you document stewardship counseling?

Individual Reflection

• What question about Doxy-PEP do you still have?

• What would make you feel safe and supported in using prevention tools?

Systems Consideration

• Does your community have consistent guidance and access pathways for Doxy-PEP?

• Are public health systems monitoring resistance patterns and outcomes?

Chapter 11

Prevention in Practice: Implementation Toolkit for Clinics, Colleges, and Health Departments

This chapter is designed for real-world implementation. It provides a toolkit for integrating prevention into routine care without increasing burden. Effective HIV and STI prevention depends on consistent implementation.

Evidence-based tools such as PrEP and Doxy-PEP are only effective when integrated into routine clinical workflows. Variability in screening, inconsistent documentation, and fragmented referral systems limit the impact of prevention (Centers for Disease Control and Prevention [CDC], 2023).

This chapter provides a structured implementation framework designed for:

- Primary care practices
- Sexual health clinics
- College health centers
- Community clinics
- Health departments

The goal is operational clarity

Step 1: Standardize Exposure-Based Screening

Prevention begins with routine screening.

Exposure-based questions should be integrated into intake forms or electronic health records (EHRs) rather than left to provider discretion.

Sample Screening Prompts

- Have you had any new sexual partners in the past six months?
- Do you know the HIV status of your partners?
- Have you had a sexually transmitted infection in the past year?
- Do you use condoms consistently?
- Do you inject drugs or share equipment?

These questions should be asked universally, not selectively.

Standardization reduces implicit bias and improves consistency.

Step 2: Create a Prevention Eligibility Pathway

Once exposure risk is identified, a clear protocol should be determined:

- PrEP eligibility
- Doxy-PEP consideration
- Vaccination review
- STI testing interval

Eligibility algorithms should be visible to staff and embedded in workflow.

Prevention discussions should be triggered by:

- Recurrent STIs
- Partner living with HIV
- Multiple partners with inconsistent condom use

- Drug Use Injection: Clear pathways prevent missed opportunities.

Step 3: Establish Monitoring Protocols

PrEP monitoring requires structured follow-up (USPSTF, 2023).

Clinics should standardize:

- Baseline HIV testing
- Renal function assessment (oral regimens)
- Quarterly HIV testing
- Routine STI screening
- Documentation of adherence discussions

Doxy-PEP protocols should include:

- Clear dosing instructions
- Frequency guidance
- Antimicrobial stewardship considerations
- Monitoring for recurrent infections

Monitoring is the prevention of integrity.

Step 4: Address Access and Navigation

Prevention uptake improves when access barriers are minimized.

Clinics should:

- Maintain updated medication assistance information
- Provide cost transparency
- Coordinate laboratory services
- Offering flexible scheduling
- Utilize telehealth when appropriate

Health departments can strengthen prevention by:

- Supporting mobile clinics
- Partnering with community organizations
- Funding navigation support roles

Navigation support reduces discontinuation.

Step 5: Normalize Prevention Conversations

Language matters.

Prevention should be framed as routine healthcare.

Instead of:
"You're high risk."

Use:
"We offer prevention options to anyone with potential exposure."

Normalization reduces stigma and increases acceptance.

Staff training should include:

- Exposure-based language
- Nonjudgmental communication
- Cultural responsiveness
- Confidentiality reinforcement

Prevention culture influences uptake.

Step 6: Integrate Layered Prevention

Clinics should avoid siloed approaches.

Prevention programs should integrate:

- HIV testing
- PrEP
- Doxy-PEP (when indicated)
- STI treatment
- Vaccination
- Harm reduction resources

Fragmentation reduces effectiveness.

Integration strengthens population-level impact.

Step 7: Measure and Evaluate

Data improves implementation.

Programs should monitor:

- PrEP uptake rates
- STI recurrence rates
- Follow-up adherence
- Discontinuation reasons
- Access disparities

Evaluation supports quality improvement.

Continuous monitoring aligns prevention with public health goals (CDC, 2023).

Sample Workflow Model

1. Patient completes standardized exposure screening.
2. Positive exposure indicators trigger prevention discussion.
3. Eligibility pathway determines PrEP and/or Doxy-PEP consideration.
4. Baseline labs obtained.
5. Medication initiated.
6. Follow-up scheduled before the patient leaves the visit.
7. Reminder system activated.
8. Access assistance provided if needed.

Structured workflow reduces variability.

Clinical Vignette

A community clinic reviews internal data and identifies that only 35% of eligible patients with recurrent STIs were offered PrEP.

The clinic implements:

- Standardized screening prompts
- Automatic EHR alerts
- Staff training on exposure-based assessment

Within six months, PrEP offering rates increase significantly.

Prevention improvement results from systems change, not medication innovation.

Implementation in College Health Settings

College populations often experience:

- New exposure patterns
- Increased STI incidence

- Variable insurance coverage

College health programs should:

- Incorporate exposure screening into annual visits
- Offer PrEP counseling proactively
- Provide confidential billing guidance
- Collaborate with campus health promotion offices

Young adults benefit from early engagement in prevention.

Implementation in Health Departments

Health departments can:

- Provide training for community clinicians
- Expand mobile testing and PrEP initiation
- Support medication assistance programs
- Integrate Doxy-PEP education where appropriate
- Use data to target high-incidence areas

Prevention impact scales when public health infrastructure aligns with clinical practice.

Chapter Summary

Prevention effectiveness depends on implementation.

Successful programs include:

- Standardized exposure-based screening
- Clear eligibility pathways
- Structured monitoring protocols
- Navigation support
- Normalized communication
- Layered prevention integration
- Ongoing evaluation

Biomedical tools reduce risk. Systems determine reach.

Reflection

Clinical Reflection

• Is your workflow prevention-ready or prevention-dependent on individual provider motivation?

• Are labs and follow-ups streamlined?

• Do you track retention and equity metrics?

Individual Reflection

• Do you know what to expect when you ask for prevention services, labs, follow-ups, and costs?

• What would make the process feel simpler?

Systems Consideration

• Are prevention programs funded and staffed to support navigation?

• Are partnerships (CBOs, colleges, health departments) leveraged effectively?

Chapter 12

The Future of Prevention: Innovation

HIV prevention has evolved significantly over the past three decades. What was once limited to behavioral counseling and condom promotion now includes highly effective biomedical tools, structured screening protocols, and integrated public health strategies.

Despite progress, HIV and bacterial STI transmission continues. The future of prevention will depend not only on new technologies but on how effectively existing tools are implemented and equitably distributed (Centers for Disease Control and Prevention [CDC], 2023; World Health Organization [WHO], 2022).

This chapter explores emerging prevention innovations and outlines priorities for the next phase of HIV and STI control.

Long-Acting Prevention Technologies

One of the most significant advancements in recent years is the development of long-acting injectable PrEP.

Long-acting cabotegravir has demonstrated high efficacy in preventing HIV acquisition and may improve adherence for individuals who struggle with daily oral medication (Landovitz et al., 2021).

Injectable Cabotegravir (Apretude)

Injectable cabotegravir is a long-acting integrase strand transfer inhibitor (INSTI) approved for HIV pre-exposure prophylaxis.

Mechanism of Action

Cabotegravir inhibits HIV integrase, preventing viral DNA from integrating into host cells.

Dosing

- Optional oral lead-in
- 600 mg intramuscular injection
- Initial two doses 1 month apart
- Maintenance dosing every 2 months

Lenacapavir: Twice-Yearly PrEP

Lenacapavir represents a next-generation long-acting prevention agent and is a first-in-class HIV capsid inhibitor.

Mechanism of Action

Lenacapavir targets the HIV-1 capsid protein, interfering with:

- Capsid assembly and disassembly
- Nuclear import
- Viral replication

This mechanism differs from both NRTIs and integrase inhibitors, offering a novel therapeutic target.

Long-acting formulations:

- Reduce daily pill burden

- Minimize reliance on patient memory
- Provide sustained drug levels
- May reduce stigma associated with pill bottles

Future research continues to explore:

- Extended-interval injectable regimens
- Implantable prevention devices
- Multipurpose prevention technologies combining contraception and HIV protection

Long-acting prevention may reduce adherence-related disparities.

Expanding STI Prevention Strategies

The introduction of Doxy-PEP represents an expansion of STI prevention beyond treatment alone (Luetkemeyer et al., 2023).

Future research priorities include:

- Refining eligibility criteria
- Monitoring antimicrobial resistance patterns
- Evaluating long-term population-level impact
- Assessing microbiome effects

Public health agencies will need to balance:

- Individual benefit
- Antimicrobial stewardship
- Resistance surveillance

The future of STI prevention will require careful integration of targeted prophylaxis within structured oversight.

Advances in HIV Treatment as Prevention

Antiretroviral therapy for people living with HIV has achieved a critical public health milestone: sustained viral suppression eliminates sexual transmission risk, a concept often summarized as "Undetectable =

Untransmittable" (U=U) (WHO, 2022).

Treatment as prevention reinforces the importance of:

- Early diagnosis
- Rapid linkage to care
- Adherence support
- Retention in care

The future of prevention integrates:

- PrEP for HIV-negative individuals
- Antiretroviral therapy for people living with HIV
- Routine testing
- Equity-driven implementation

Transmission declines when both prevention and treatment are optimized

Data-Driven Public Health Approaches

Surveillance data increasingly guide prevention strategies.

Modern prevention frameworks use:

- Geographic incidence mapping
- Real-time STI reporting
- Community viral load data
- Program evaluation metrics

Data allows:

- Targeted outreach
- Resource allocation
- Identification of underserved areas
- Measurement of intervention impact

However, data must be interpreted within context. Surveillance reflects both access and exposure patterns.

Data-informed prevention improves precision.

Equity as a Central Priority

Persistent disparities indicate that prevention tools are not reaching all populations equally (CDC, 2023).

Future progress depends on:

- Expanding access in rural regions
- Reducing insurance barriers
- Integrating culturally responsive care
- Addressing stigma at institutional levels
- Strengthening community partnerships

Innovation without equity widens disparities.

The next phase of prevention must prioritize access as strongly as technology.

Integrating Prevention into Primary Care

Historically, HIV prevention was often delivered through specialty clinics.

The future requires:

- Normalization within primary care
- Integration into routine wellness visits
- Inclusion in college health programs
- Standardized exposure screening across settings

Prevention should not require referral to specialized centers unless clinically necessary.

Decentralization improves reach.

The Role of Telehealth and Digital Health

Telehealth expansion has increased access to prevention services, particularly in areas with provider shortages.

Digital tools may support:

- Remote PrEP initiation
- Laboratory coordination
- Adherence reminders
- Patient education
- Appointment scheduling

However, digital access disparities must be addressed to prevent widening inequities.

Technology is a facilitator, not a substitute for access infrastructure

A Future-Oriented Clinical Vignette

A community health center integrates:

- Standardized exposure screening
- Same-day PrEP initiation
- Doxy-PEP eligibility protocols
- Telehealth follow-up
- Data-driven quality improvement tracking

Within two years, new HIV diagnoses decline, and recurrent STI rates stabilize.

The change did not require breakthroughs in medication.

It required a structured implementation.

The future of prevention may depend less on discovery and more on integration.

Prevention as a Dynamic Model

Prevention strategies will continue to evolve.

Future directions may include:

- Vaccine development
- Extended-release antiretrovirals
- Combination prevention platforms
- Artificial intelligence–guided risk assessment
- Expanded harm reduction models

Adaptability will be essential. Prevention must remain:

- Evidence-based
- Exposure-focused
- Equity-driven

- Integrated across systems

Closing Message

Prevention is not about fear. It's about power, giving people options, information, and support to protect their health without judgment.

Chapter Summary

The future of HIV and STI prevention depends on:

- Expanding long-acting technologies
- Responsible integration of Doxy-PEP
- Strengthening treatment-as-prevention
- Using data to guide interventions
- Prioritizing equity
- Integrating prevention into routine care
- Leveraging digital health tools responsibly

Biomedical innovation is important.

But sustained impact will depend on structured implementation and equitable access.

Prevention works when systems support it.

Table 1A. Dosing and Administration of HIV PrEP Options

Feature	Daily Oral PrEP	Injectable PrEP (Cabotegravir)	Extended-Interval PrEP(Lenacapavir / Yeztugo®)
Route of Administration	Oral tablet	Intramuscular injection	Subcutaneous injection
Dosing Frequency	Daily	Every 2 months	Every 6 months (twice yearly)
Medication Class	NRTI-based	Integrase inhibitor	Capsid inhibitor
Adherence Requirement	Daily pill adherence	Clinic visit every 2 months	Clinic visit twice yearly

Table 1B. Clinical Use and Considerations

Feature	Daily Oral PrEP	Injectable PrEP	Extended-Interval PrEP
FDA Approval Status	Approved	Approved	FDA-approved for HIV PrEP
Ideal Candidates	Comfortable with daily meds	Difficulty with daily adherence	Prefer minimal dosing frequency
Key Advantages	Widely available	Eliminates daily pills	Longest dosing interval
Key Considerations	Daily adherence	Injection site reactions	Cost, access, long pharmacologic tail
Role in Prevention	Foundational option	Long-acting alternative	Extended-interval option

81

Reflection

Clinical Reflection

• What innovation could most improve prevention in your setting: long-acting options, better navigation, or integrated services?

• Are your systems ready to adopt new prevention tools without increasing inequities?

Individual Reflection

• What prevention option feels most aligned with your life right now?

• What support would help you take the next step?

Systems Consideration

• How will your community ensure new prevention tools are distributed equitably?

• What metrics will define success beyond prescriptions (retention, outcomes, reduced disparities)?

• Are emerging technologies equitably distributed?

• Are surveillance data used to reduce disparities?

• Is prevention integrated across healthcare settings?

Appendix A:

Clinical Laboratory Quick Reference Guide for PrEP Care

This quick reference guide summarizes commonly recommended laboratory tests for initiating and monitoring pre-exposure prophylaxis (PrEP). These evaluations help ensure patient safety, confirm HIV-negative status, and support comprehensive sexual health care.

PrEP Initiation: Baseline Laboratory Evaluation

Before starting PrEP, clinicians should confirm HIV-negative status and assess renal function, hepatitis status, and sexually transmitted infections.

HIV Testing

- HIV antigen/antibody (4th generation) with reflex confirmation
- HIV viral load (HIV RNA PCR) if acute infection is suspected (e.g., recent high-risk exposure, symptoms of seroconversion)
- **HIV viral load (HIV RNA PCR) is recommended prior to initiation of long-acting injectable PrEP (e.g., cabotegravir, lenacapavir) to reduce the risk of initiating therapy during undiagnosed acute HIV infection**

Sexually Transmitted Infection Screening

- **Gonorrhea and Chlamydia NAAT testing**
  - Urine or vaginal swab
  - Throat swab (based on exposure)

- o Rectal swab (based on exposure)
- **Syphilis screening**
    - o RPR with reflex titer and confirmatory testing

Hepatitis Screening

- Hepatitis B panel
    - o Hepatitis B surface antigen
    - o Hepatitis B surface antibody
    - o Hepatitis B core antibody
- Hepatitis A antibody (total) if vaccination status unknown
- Hepatitis C antibody with reflex quantitative testing

Renal Function

- Basic metabolic panel (BMP)
- Serum creatinine
- Blood urea nitrogen (BUN)

Pregnancy Testing

- Serum hCG (if pregnancy is possible)

Baseline testing ensures that patients are appropriate candidates for PrEP therapy and allows clinicians to identify coexisting infections that require treatment.

PrEP Follow-Up Monitoring

Patients receiving PrEP should be monitored regularly to ensure continued HIV-negative status, medication safety, and ongoing sexual health counseling.

Every 3 Months

- HIV antigen/antibody test with reflex confirmation

- STI screening
  - Gonorrhea and Chlamydia (urine, throat, rectal as indicated)
  - Syphilis (RPR with reflex titer and confirmation)
- Adherence counseling
- Risk-reduction counseling

Every 6–12 Months

- Renal function monitoring
  - Serum creatinine
  - Blood urea nitrogen (BUN)
  - Basic metabolic panel as indicated

As Clinically Indicated

- Pregnancy testing
- Hepatitis monitoring
- Additional STI testing based on symptoms or exposure risk

Clinical Pearl

Routine laboratory monitoring supports safe PrEP prescribing and strengthens comprehensive HIV prevention strategies by identifying early infections, minimizing the risk of initiating PrEP during undiagnosed acute HIV infection, and ensuring ongoing patient engagement in care.

HIV RNA & Long-Acting PrEP

Chapter 13

The Future of HIV Prevention: Extended-Interval and Adherence-Independent Strategies

Introduction

HIV prevention has evolved dramatically over the past decade. What began as daily oral pre-exposure prophylaxis (PrEP) has expanded to include long-acting injectable agents, post-exposure strategies for preventing bacterial STIs, and emerging extended-interval innovations. The trajectory of prevention science reflects a broader public health goal: reducing reliance on daily adherence and minimizing structural barriers to protection.

The future of HIV prevention lies in strategies that are durable, discreet, equitable, and adaptable to diverse populations.

Moving Beyond Daily Adherence

Daily oral PrEP remains highly effective when taken consistently, reducing sexual HIV acquisition risk by approximately 99% (Centers for Disease Control and Prevention [CDC], 2023). However, adherence challenges persist due to:

- Stigma
- Housing instability
- Pill fatigue
- Medical mistrust
- Limited healthcare access
- Privacy concerns

Long-acting and extended-interval agents represent a paradigm shift by decreasing the behavioral burden placed on patients. Instead of requiring daily action, prevention becomes event-based, clinic-based, or biannual.

This shift reframes prevention from daily responsibility to a structured medical intervention.

Injectable Prevention as the New Standard

Long-acting injectable cabotegravir demonstrated superiority over daily oral PrEP in major clinical trials (Landovitz et al., 2021; Delany-Moretlwe et al., 2022). Its implementation signals a move toward adherence-independent protection models.

Twice-yearly agents, such as lenacapavir, further advance this evolution by potentially reducing prevention dosing to only two injections per year.

Extended-interval prevention may:

- Increase uptake among adolescents and young adults
- Improve prevention equity in marginalized communities
- Reduce stigma associated with visible daily medication
- Simplify public health delivery models

As dosing intervals lengthen, prevention becomes less intrusive and more sustainable.

Integration of STI Prevention Strategies

The addition of doxycycline post-exposure prophylaxis (Doxy-PEP) introduces another layer of modern sexual health protection. Clinical trials demonstrate significant reductions in syphilis and chlamydia incidence among high-risk populations (Luetkemeyer et al., 2023).

Future prevention models will likely integrate:

- HIV PrEP
- Doxy-PEP
- Routine STI screening
- Vaccination strategies
- Behavioral risk reduction counseling

The movement toward combination prevention reflects recognition that sexual health is multidimensional.

Equity and Structural Considerations

Scientific advancement alone does not eliminate disparities. The communities most impacted by HIV, including Black and Hispanic populations, LGBTQ+ individuals, and those in the Southern United States, continue to face disproportionate barriers to prevention access (U.S. Department of Health and Human Services, 2024).

Future prevention efforts must prioritize:

- Insurance coverage expansion
- Community-based delivery models
- Culturally responsive care
- Reduction of stigma in healthcare settings
- Provider education

Biomedical innovation must be paired with structural reform.

Pipeline and Emerging Technologies

Beyond currently available long-acting injectables, the
prevention pipeline includes:

- Capsid inhibitors with extended durability
- Broadly neutralizing antibodies
- Long-acting implants
- Multipurpose prevention technologies
- Combination HIV and STI injectable platforms

These innovations aim to further reduce dosing frequency,
enhance tolerability, and expand protection options across
diverse patient populations.

As these agents mature through clinical development, providers
must remain adaptable and informed.

The Role of the Clinician

Modern HIV prevention demands more than prescribing
medication. It requires:

- Risk assessment expertise
- Cultural humility
- Shared decision-making
- Routine HIV and STI screening
- Education on evolving prevention modalities

Clinicians must present prevention options as personalized,
evidence-based choices rather than one-size-fits-all solutions.

A Prevention-Centered Public Health Model

The future of HIV prevention aligns with national Ending the HIV Epidemic initiatives aimed at reducing new infections by 90% (U.S. Department of Health and Human Services, 2024).

To reach this goal, prevention must become:

- Routine
- Accessible
- Normalized
- Integrated into primary care
- Supported by policy and funding

Extended-interval prevention strategies may significantly accelerate progress toward epidemic control.

Conclusion

HIV prevention is no longer limited to daily oral medication. It is an evolving landscape characterized by innovation, flexibility, and expanding choice.

From daily PrEP to injectable cabotegravir, from Doxy-PEP to twice-yearly lenacapavir, prevention science continues to advance toward models that reduce adherence burden and increase equity.

The future of HIV prevention is:

- Longer acting
- Less stigmatizing
- More personalized
- More accessible

*As biomedical tools advance, healthcare professionals'
responsibility is to ensure these innovations reach the
populations who need them most.*

Modern HIV prevention is not simply about medication.
It is about implementation, equity, and sustained commitment to
ending the epidemic.

Final Reflection

A Commitment to Prevention

HIV prevention has never been solely about medication. It has always been about access, education, dignity, and equity.

Throughout my career, I have witnessed both the extraordinary progress of biomedical science and the persistent gaps that leave vulnerable communities at risk. We now have tools that previous generations of clinicians could only imagine: daily oral PrEP, long-acting injectable agents, Doxy-PEP, and emerging extended-interval prevention strategies. These innovations have transformed what is possible.

Yet despite these advances, preventable infections continue to occur.

This reality reinforces a central truth: science alone is not enough. Implementation matters. Access matters. Trust matters.

My passion for HIV prevention grew from witnessing preventable infections in young adults and underserved communities, reinforcing the importance of proactive, informed prevention strategies. Many of these individuals had limited access to care, faced stigma, or were simply unaware of the options available to protect themselves. Prevention must therefore extend beyond prescription pads and clinical guidelines. It must be embedded in community education, culturally responsive care, and policy-level commitment.

Modern HIV prevention is not about replacing one medication with another. It is about expanding choice. Some patients prefer daily oral protection. Others benefit from an injectable regimen. Some may utilize Doxy-PEP as part of comprehensive sexual health planning. The role of the clinician is to guide, educate, and individualize prevention strategies in ways that respect autonomy and lived experience.

The future of HIV prevention is promising. Extended-interval injectables, capsid inhibitors, and combination prevention technologies may further reduce barriers and improve adherence. However, the true measure of progress will not be found in clinical trial data alone. It will be reflected in reduced disparities, increased uptake among marginalized populations, and sustained declines in new HIV diagnoses.

Ending the HIV epidemic requires sustained commitment from clinicians, public health leaders, policymakers, and communities alike.

As healthcare professionals, we have the privilege and responsibility to translate scientific advancement into meaningful protection for those we serve.

Prevention is not simply a clinical intervention.

It is a commitment.

References

American Academy of HIV Medicine. (2023). *Clinical resources for HIV care and prevention.* American Academy of HIV Medicine. https://aahivm.org

American Academy of HIV Medicine. (2025). *HIV specialist clinical reference guide* (2025 ed.). American Academy of HIV Medicine.

Baeten, J. M., Donnell, D., Ndase, P., Mugo, N. R., Campbell, J. D., Wangisi, J., Tappero, J. W., Bukusi, E. A., Cohen, C. R., Katabira, E., Ronald, A., Tumwesigye, E., Were, E., Fife, K. H., Kiarie, J., Farquhar, C., John-Stewart, G., Kakia, A., Odoyo, J., & Celum, C. (2012). Antiretroviral prophylaxis for HIV prevention in heterosexual men and women. *New England Journal of Medicine, 367*(5), 399–410. https://doi.org/10.1056/NEJMoa1108524

Centers for Disease Control and Prevention. (2021). *Sexually transmitted infections treatment guidelines, 2021.* U.S. Department of Health and Human Services. https://www.cdc.gov/std/treatment

Centers for Disease Control and Prevention. (2023). *Preexposure prophylaxis for the prevention of HIV infection in the United States—2023 update: A clinical practice guideline.* U.S. Department of Health and Human Services. https://www.cdc.gov/hiv

Centers for Disease Control and Prevention. (2024). *HIV prevention: Pre-exposure prophylaxis (PrEP).* https://www.cdc.gov/hiv/prevention/prep

Cohen, M. S., Molina, J. M., & Cates, W. (2024). New directions in HIV prevention: Long-acting agents and emerging strategies. *The Lancet HIV, 11*(1), e1–e3. https://doi.org/10.1016/S2352-3018(23)00245-8

Gilead Sciences, Inc. (2023). *Descovy® (emtricitabine and tenofovir alafenamide) prescribing information.* Gilead Sciences, Inc. https://www.gilead.com

Gilead Sciences, Inc. (2023). *Truvada® (emtricitabine and tenofovir disoproxil fumarate) prescribing information.* Gilead Sciences, Inc. https://www.gilead.com

Gilead Sciences, Inc. (2024). *HIV prevention and PrEP clinical resources.* Gilead Sciences, Inc. https://www.gilead.com

Grant, R. M., Anderson, P. L., McMahan, V., Liu, A. Y., Amico, K. R., Mehrotra, M., Hosek, S., Mosquera, C., Casapia, M., Montoya-Herrera, O., Buchbinder, S., Veloso, V. G., Mayer, K. H., & Glidden, D. V. (2014). Uptake of pre-exposure prophylaxis, sexual practices, and HIV incidence in men and transgender women who have sex with men: A cohort study. *The Lancet Infectious Diseases, 14*(9), 820–829. https://doi.org/10.1016/S1473-3099(14)70847-3

Grant, R. M., Lama, J. R., Anderson, P. L., McMahan, V., Liu, A. Y., Vargas, L., Goicochea, P., Casapía, M., Guanira-Carranza, J. V., Ramirez-Cardich, M. E., Montoya-Herrera, O., Fernández, T., Veloso, V. G., Buchbinder, S. P., Chariyalertsak, S., Schechter, M., Bekker, L. G., Mayer, K. H., Kallás, E. G., & Glidden, D. V. (2010). Preexposure chemoprophylaxis for HIV prevention in men who have sex with men. *New England Journal of Medicine, 363*(27), 2587–2599. https://doi.org/10.1056/NEJMoa1011205

HIV Medicine Association. (2022). *Primary care guidance for persons with HIV.* Infectious Diseases Society of America. https://www.idsociety.org

Luetkemeyer, A. F., Donnell, D., Dombrowski, J. C., Cohen, S. E., Grabow, C., Brown, C. E., et al. (2023). Doxycycline postexposure prophylaxis for bacterial sexually transmitted infections. *New England Journal of Medicine, 388*(14), 1296–1306. https://doi.org/10.1056/NEJMoa2211934

McCormack, S., Dunn, D. T., Desai, M., Dolling, D. I., Gafos, M., Gilson, R., Sullivan, A. K., Clarke, A., Reeves, I., Schembri, G., Mackie, N., Bowman, C., Lacey, C. J., Apea, V., Brady, M., Fox, J., Taylor, S., Antonucci, S., Khoo, S., & Gill, O. N. (2016). Pre-exposure prophylaxis to prevent the acquisition of HIV-1 infection (PROUD): Effectiveness results from the pilot phase of a pragmatic open-label randomised trial. *The Lancet, 387*(10013), 53–60. https://doi.org/10.1016/S0140-6736(15)00056-2

Molina, J. M., Charreau, I., Chidiac, C., Pialoux, G., Cua, E., Delaugerre, C., et al. (2018). Post-exposure doxycycline to prevent sexually transmitted infections in men who have sex with men: An open-label randomized substudy of the ANRS IPERGAY trial. *The Lancet Infectious Diseases, 18*(3), 308–317. https://doi.org/10.1016/S1473-3099(17)30725-9

National Institutes of Health. (2023). *Guidelines for the use of antiretroviral agents in adults and adolescents with HIV.* U.S. Department of Health and Human Services. https://clinicalinfo.hiv.gov

U.S. Preventive Services Task Force. (2023). Preexposure prophylaxis for the prevention of HIV infection: Preventive medication. *JAMA, 329*(7), 592–598. https://doi.org/10.1001/jama.2022.21949

World Health Organization. (2022). *Consolidated guidelines on HIV prevention, testing, treatment, service delivery and monitoring.* World Health Organization. https://www.who.int

World Health Organization. (2023). *HIV prevention, diagnosis, treatment and care for key populations.* World Health Organization. https://www.who.int

www.ingramcontent.com/pod-product-compliance
Lightning Source LLC
Chambersburg PA
CBHW022129150726
47991CB00008B/3135